I0426328

Paleo Diet For Beginners

What is Paleo Diet, Health Benefits, Allowed Food List And Lose Weight

By: Russell Dawson

ISBN :978-1491269534

TABLE OF CONTENTS

PUBLISHERS NOTES

Disclaimer

DEDICATION

Dedicated with love to my family.

Chapter 1 - Introduction

Our modern society is beleaguered with a lot of health problems that can be ascribed to obesity as well as improper and poor diet. According to O'Keefe et. al. (2011), this present situation is largely because our daily physical activities in this technological age greatly differ from what our genes has been designed for. The natural environment requiring various physical activities for survival that humans used to inhabit has long been gone. The physically demanding environment our ancestors lived in has now been replaced by cities with elevators, escalators, bullet trains, airplanes, quick modes of transportation, fast-food counters, supermarket chains, and electronic banking systems.

Logically, the solution is to provide the human activity patterns our bodies and genes have been designed for in a manner that is practical and achievable in our modern environment. This will involve more rigorous exercise routines and activities to simulate the more physically demanding lifestyle of our ancestors who were hunters, gatherers, warriors, and trades people.

There are many types of diets human beings have adopted through the years, ranging from omnivorous, vegetarian, combination diets, diets for a beautiful body, diets for health, diets for an athletic lifestyle, and other lifestyle diets. In the old days, diets evolved because inhabitants have to adapt to the limited offerings of nature, the earth, and its seasons. In the modern world, humans can choose diets according to their needs, and their beliefs as the supply of food is no longer limited by the season, topography, available arable land, and the number of family and clan members providing food.

Humans progressively learned to hunt, to gather from the wild, to make fire, to plant crops, to care for animals, to keep herds, to propagate plants and animals for food, to trade and barter, to boost food production, and to process food so that its availability will not be dependent on the seasons. Ultimately, new technology led to new products and processes with the use of newly discovered processes, chemicals and additives. Consequently, humans began to be beleaguered with chronic diseases and health problems.

Scholars and health gurus began their research into these chronic diseases plaguing the modern world and in the 1970s came up with the theory that the genetic disposition of man is not meant to eat processed foods and foods that are not from nature. The Paleo Diet was born out of this theory. Paleo is short for the word Paleolithic, and thus it aims to recreate the diet of the Paleolithic man, claiming that it is the diet and the lifestyle the human body has been designed for.

The Paleo Diet is proposed as the solution for the health problems of the modern man, as our Paleolithic ancestors, aside from being killed young in battle or as a hunter, lived long, healthy lives. They were robust, strong, active, energetic, tough, and powerful. Therefore, it is proposed that modern man look back to the ways and diet of its Paleolithic ancestors and eat as they ate..

CHAPTER 2- WHAT IS PALEO DIET-THE BASICS

The Paleo diet (also known as the Paleolithic- diet) is a type of 'modern nutritional plan based an alleged ancient diet of wild plant and animals, consumed by various hominid species during the Paleolithic era over 2.5 million years ago.' This diet soon developed into modern human diets upon the development of agricultural and grain-based produce.

Also known as the caveman diet, this contemporary version of the early Paleo diet consists of fish, grass-fed meats, eggs, fruits and vegetables, fungi, roots and nuts. The diet, however, excludes legumes, dairy products, potatoes, refined salts and sugars, in addition to processed oils.

The main concept of this diet revolves around the assumption that 'modern humans are genetically adapted to their Paleolithic ancestral diet, since human genetics have changed little since the introduction of agriculture to the modern world.' As a result of this theory, many Paleo experts assume that the 'ideal diet for human health is a diet best resembling the Paleo diet.'

Behind the Paleo Diet

The Paleo 'way of eating' is spreading to people from all walks of life. As people transitioned to modern diets containing grains and dairy from their agricultural efforts, the rise of cardiovascular and other inflammatory diseases seemed to start affecting people most susceptible to the conditions. These people also happened to consume modern diets with grains and dairy.

Research indicates that modern hunter-gatherer societies actually experience less harmful symptoms found with modern diets in first world societies. This indicates that the hunter-gatherer way of eating (the Paleo diet) may be suitable for people wanting to avoid contracting symptoms from various cardiovascular and similar conditions.

People on the Paleo diet have experienced results amounting to: significant weight loss, muscle gain, increases in their energy reserves, less inflammation from various conditions and an overall sense of rejuvenation in both skin and the rest of the body. People with gastrointestinal problems may also benefit from this diet, due to the lack of problematic foods that don't easily digest like dairy.

Even people with diabetes may benefit from this diet; some diabetes sufferers actually experience symptoms that make them less dependent on their insulin medication. Anyone with a debilitating condition like diabetes, however, should always consult their doctor for advice before changing their dieting habits.

The Paleo diet provides great 'framework' for people who want to lose weight by cutting foods that may not digest well in their bodies. People who also want to get more fit also benefit from this diet, too. Becoming closer with our ancestral origins naturally involves bringing food into the picture—and the Paleo diet is one of those ways that also makes us more healthier as a result.

. The basis of the Paleo Diet is the main diet of mankind's ancestors during the Paleolithic era. As grains such as oats, rice, and wheat were only introduced around 10,000 years ago, they are not included in the foods to be eaten. The wheat free and grain free Paleo Diet is composed mainly of lean meats, fish, seeds, fresh fruits, vegetables, eggs, healthful oils, and nuts.

The Paleo Diet is based upon the consumption of wholesome foods that our hunter-gatherer ancestors used to eat during the Paleolithic era. It is basically eating only foods that can be made available for consumption without the use of technology except for a stone or sharp stick. Cereal grains, potatoes, legumes, dairy products, processed foods, and refined sugars were non-existent in the Paleolithic era.

Hunter-gatherers were generally free from chronic diseases and illnesses that are prevalent in our modern populations such as cardiovascular diseases, stroke, congestive heart failure, heart disease, high blood pressure, atherosclerosis , obesity, type 2 diabetes, cancer, multiple sclerosis, Chrohn's disease, rheumatoid arthritis, ulcerative colitis, other autoimmune diseases, osteoporosis, acne, macular degeneration, glaucoma, myopia, hemorrhoids, gastric reflux, diverticulosis, varicose veins, and gout.

The foods our ancestors consumed before the Agricultural Revolution hundreds of generations ago are high in nutrients that are beneficial to the body such as antioxidants, phytochemicals, soluble fiber, low-glycemic carbohydrates, vitamins, omega-3, and monounsaturated fats. Paleo Diet foods promote good health and are free from additives and chemicals that may cause harm to the body.

.

CHAPTER 3- HUMAN CONSUMPTION, THE BASICS OF HUMAN NUTRITION, DIET GENERATION AND OUR OVERWEIGHT SOCIETY

Recent literature about the study of diseases plaguing our modern civilization points to the fundamental changes in human diet and the modern lifestyle that man has progressively adopted. As a consequence, a mismatch between the human physiology and the modern diet now exists which has been blamed for lifestyle diseases of the modern world such as obesity, diabetes, hypertension, coronary heart disease, epithelial cell cancers and osteoporosis. These diseases were non-existent in the ancient generations when our ancestors hunted extensively to provide food for their clans as well as cultivated and gathered crops (Carrera-Bastos, et. al., 2011). Therefore, it has been proposed that man's diets and lifestyle should be modified to adopt those of the pre-agricultural environment as a way of reducing the risks and preventing the onset of chronic degenerative diseases.

According to a Global Health Observatory (2011) article published in the World Health Organization website, an approximate 16.0 million disability adjusted life years (DALYs) and 1.7 million of global deaths are attributed to low consumption of fruit and vegetables. Studies showed that high energy high-fat processed food consumption promotes obesity while adequate consumption of low-energy foods like fruits and vegetables can help reduce the risk of stomach cancer, colorectal cancer, and cardiovascular diseases.

The WHO recommends a low salt intake of less than 5 grams per day per person to prevent cardiovascular disease and high blood pressure. Heart disease has also been linked to high consumption of trans-fatty acids and saturated fats, so the use of polyunsaturated vegetable oils is recommended to lower the risks not only of coronary heart disease but also of type 2 diabetes.

In a study conducted by the Jean Mayer Human Nutrition Research Center on Aging at Tufts University in Boston and published by the Agricultural Research Service of the U. S. Department of Agriculture, it was found that plasma antioxidant capacity in humans can increase with a diet high in fruits and vegetables. The study was conducted with 36 healthy non-smokers. The subjects stayed in a metabolic research unit and were grouped into two. One group consumed a controlled diet of fruits and vegetables for 15 days. The other group received the same diet except for an additional 2 servings of broccoli from day 6-10. The oxygen radical absorbance capacity (ORAC) of the subjects was measured as well as alpha-tocopherol concentrations on specific days. The fasting plasma oxidant capacity of the subjects taking both types of diets increased significantly.

Humans were largely vegetarian during most of man's evolutionary history. In ancient times, plant foods and tubers made up most of the human diet. When fire was discovered, humans started to eat more meat. Early humans needed the nourishment from meat because there were seasons when plant foods were scarce or unavailable. Centuries ago, meats were only for the wealthiest people. Serfs and ordinary people feed the livestock and raise them for their masters but they seldom get their share of offal and leftovers. As a consequence, only the rich people suffered from obesity and heart disease before the 20th century. These days, animal flesh is easily available and relatively affordable, so the per capita consumption of meat has doubled since the 1950s. In direct proportion, the cases of deadly ailments such as cancer, stroke, and heart disease have become common complaints.

As humans started to eat less fruits, nuts, and leaves and consumed more meat, their brains grew. The development of tools enabled humans to hunt for food which they were able to cook with fire. There was no longer a need for sharp, big teeth and big grinders to deal with uncut raw meat. These changes in eating habits were evident in human skulls uncovered in various anthropological sites dating back to millions of years ago.

Man's early diet of fruits, nuts, berries, roots was a low-calorie diet, so they ate a lot to obtain the needed energy and had big stomachs to accommodate the huge volume of foods. When man started to eat meat, the energy from the calories and fat went to brain development. The big guts shrank and the body built up the brain, so men learned to make better tools and became smarter. Human skulls, teeth, jaws, and mouth changed in accordance with the change in eating habits.

A featured article in the Centers for Disease Control and Prevention, said that fats are essential for the body to function normally, but some fats are better for human health than other fats. Cholesterol, saturated fats and trans-fats are the less healthy fats while monounsaturated fats and polyunsaturated fats are better for human consumption.

According to the 2010 Dietary Guidelines for Americans, Americans should eat less saturated fat and replace solid fats in their foods with oils whenever possible. Consumption of foods containing hydrogenated oils and other trans-fatty acids should be limited or kept as low as possible. Dietary cholesterol intake should also be limited to

300 mg per day. Total fat intake should be kept between 20 to 35% of daily total calories.

Human beings have dietary needs in order to survive. Nutrients for human needs are derived from the diet. Humans need calories from food for energy. There are nine essential amino acids that the body needs for the synthesis of protein. There are three essential fatty acids that the body needs for its functions. The body needs 18 different minerals in varying amounts as well as various vitamins that are all sourced from food.

There is still much debate in the determination of what substances are really essential for survival and substances needed for general good health. Through the years, humans have recognized deficiency diseases such as scurvy for lack of Vitamin C, beriberi for lack of Vitamin B1, and pellagra for lack of niacin. However it took outbreaks of these diseases and some serious study before the deficiencies were related to the disease. When people were fed synthetic diets through intravenous feeding, physicians and medical practitioners found that trace mineral deficiencies in chromium and molybdenum of the synthetic diets resulted in some health issues (Kimball, 2011).

There are guidelines on the recommended daily allowances or RDAs of various food groups published by the Food and Nutrition Board of the U.S. National Academy of Sciences. These RDAs are found on nutrition labels of food products.

. The average person will find out if he is under weight or overweight using the body mass index or BMI. Body fat is measured by BMI based on the individual's weight and height, although this measurement is not applicable for body builders. For men and women aged 18-65 a

BMI between 20 and 25 is a healthy weight score. Other body weight scores or categories include obese, overweight, and underweight.

Obese and overweight are terms that describe individuals who weighs more than what is regarded healthy in proportion to his/her height. The BMI results serve as a guide as some healthy people may have conditions that are weight responsive. The BMI of growing children and adolescents are also plotted with their age and sex on growth charts.

Diet Generation is the creation of a daily menu that calculates the calorie intake according to an individual's body mass index. A diet generator ensures that the diet is healthy and that it will promote weight loss by releasing fat burning hormones after eating. Losing weight can also be accomplished by eating small meals in short intervals in the course of a single day. A diet plan is actually a way of eating and a way of life for some. It is designed for losing excess pounds and at the same time maintaining the achieved desired healthy weight.

The diet generation also refers to the present preoccupation, even of teen agers and adolescents with diet programs. The following as some tips that will help you to stick to a diet program.

• Regularly monitor your weight loss and/or gain. Get a weighing scale for your bathroom, so you can step on it every day.

• Be aware of your eating schedule. Wear a watch so you will remember what time you last ate your meal and know the specific intervals between your meals.

• Begin your day with a shake or a meal rich in protein.

- Do some form of exercises everyday, even if you don't go to a gym. Do some stretches, jogging or brisk walking every morning.

- Remember to eat at regular intervals, with small meals or snacks like mixed nuts, healthy sandwiches, and some of fruits or vegetables.

- Buy some protein bars and nuts to tide you over when you get too hungry before the next meal.

- Small snacks and meals help in speeding up the body's metabolism, resulting in weight loss.

- Your weight goals should be reasonable and attainable. Do not go on crash diets.

- Large meals will slow down your metabolism. Never eat a meal larger than the size of your fist, as this is roughly the size of your stomach.

- Watch and limit your carbohydrate intake. Eat more protein-rich foods.

- Keep in mind that food is needed energy for your body, it is not a reward. Eat only what your body needs.

Our Overweight Society

An article published in the Guardian said that according to a recent study, out of ten men, eight will be overweight by 2020. In the case of women, seven out of ten will also be obese by 2020. The report also showed that the incidence of heart disease, stroke and diabetes will increase accordingly. There are no signs to show that obesity cases will decrease among adults, so the report concluded that the incidence of heart disease and other obesity associated illnesses will also rise.

The new predictions were based on a study conducted by a group from Oxford University, led by Professor Klim McPherson who chairs the National Heart Forum, based on figures from 1993 to 2007. The study was undertaken for the purpose of predicting England's future obesity levels.

The report further predicts that by 2050 obesity-related stroke will increase by 23%, obesity-related high blood pressure will increase by 34%, obesity-related coronary heart disease will rise by 44%, and obesity-related diabetes incidence will rise by 98%. Professor McPherson further said that people are being overwhelmed by an overweight society, where energy-dense food is abundant and lifestyles have become sedentary.

According to Joe Korner, a director at The Stroke Association, obese people can do something about being more than a statistic and reduce the risk of having a stroke by eating more healthy foods and exercising regularly. Similarly, some key recommendations from the Dietary Guide to Americans to prevent obesity and reduce overweight include improving eating and behaviors related to physical activity. Another recommendation is the control of total calorie intake which means choosing foods and beverages with fewer calories. Finally, it is recommended that appropriate calorie balance be maintained by people in all stages of life – in childhood and adolescence, pregnancy, breastfeeding, adulthood, and old age.

A person's body weight has been proven to be affected not only by genetic factors but by environmental and behavioral factors. Calorie balance – the relationship between calories from food consumption and calories expended through metabolism and physical activities – is the key to weight management over time.

People have no control over the body's metabolic processes but they can manage their eating and drinking habits as well as their physical activities to expend excess calories. Weight gain is most often due to excess calorie consumption. In the same manner, when physical activities use up more calories than is being consumed, the result is weight loss. Over time, reduction of calorie intake or more rigorous physical activities, or both can result in weight loss and better health.

According to reports, calorie imbalance is prevalent in many American citizens. Some studies call the present situation as an obesity epidemic, because the prevalence of obesity has dramatically increased from the 1970s to 2008. Ultimately, because obesity is associated with many diseases and health conditions, it can increase individual health risks including premature death. Preventing the onset of obesity in childhood is one of the important strategies in the fight against obesity epidemic. A health care provider should be regularly consulted as they can help in the proper weight management of children and adolescents.

It has been recommended that families, communities, and schools be involved and support the change in eating habits and behaviors of children and adolescents towards physical activities. It has also been recommended that Americans of all age brackets should choose a healthy eating pattern by eating nutrient-dense foods as well as the beverages they like to meet their nutritional requirements while staying within a calorie balance. American adults should also avoid a sedentary lifestyle and be more physically active.

.Unified Field Theory.

An article written by Professor Ssali (1996) describes disease as any type of disorder or abnormality in bodily functions which maybe congenital and hereditary, the result of degenerative change in the cells of the body, or due to fungal, viral, or bacterial infection. According to Professor Ssali, diseases are traceable to some form of nutritional deficit and can be eliminated if the subject is fed a properly balanced diet from its fetal development.

Nutrients from food produce scavengers of harmful free radicals that are the products of body metabolism. Free radicals are harmful to the body and may disrupt normal fetal development. When the intake of nutrients is not enough, the body weakens and gets invaded by fungus, viruses and bacteria. Therefore, congenital abnormalities and developmental aberration can be traced back to improper nutrition. In many cases, even if the food intake is nutritious, use of drugs and toxic substances affect the cell division of the fetus that may result in congenital defects and abnormalities.

Antibodies such as lymphocytes and macrophages produced by the immune system to fight infection are also dependent on nutrition. When the body is deficient in nutrients, the immune system weakens and the body is invaded by harmful bacteria, fungus, and viruses. Nutrients provide the body with free-radical fighting antioxidants that attack abnormal and diseased cell structures. The cells regenerate when there are adequate nutrients, curing the body of illnesses and potential health problems.

Drinking lots of water is necessary in the fight against free radicals as the kidneys need help in excreting impurities. A body without adequate water supply will rapidly deteriorate due to dehydration and toxic impurities that can accumulate. Nutritional deficit and lack of water is also a major contributor to the aging process. A people age, the cells in the body fail to reproduce when the body gets dehydrated and deprived of nutrients such as vitamins and minerals.

Nutrients fail to be utilized by the body when there are toxic substances from the internal and external environment that blocks their beneficial effects. This explains why the incidence of cancer increases with age - due to accumulation of toxins over the years. Taking contraceptives, abuse of antibiotics, and cigarette smoking are just some of the factors that contribute to the increase of toxins in the body. Those laden with toxins have greater risk of developing cancer of the prostate, lungs, uterus, and breast.

The detoxification of free radicals is a response of the immune system which results in nutritional deficit. A body that is nutritionally deficient develops chronic diseases like high blood pressure, asthma, and diabetes. A nutritious diet and plenty of water helps keep the health of the body close to ideal for a long time. Antioxidants from the consumption of fresh fruit and vegetables mop up the harmful free radicals in the body, thereby eliminating the disease causing virus and cancer cells. The immune system gets the strength to protect the body from nutrient- rich foods.

The body's immune system is so powerful but this power is largely dependent on the nutrients it gets regularly. Many viruses only manifest their presence when the body is malnourished and deficient in nutrients. Cancer cells start to develop because the natural killer cells that fight them are weakened by poor nutrition. Oftentimes, a person who eats sufficient amounts of nutritious food lose the nutrients because they were used up by the body to get rid of toxic substances also ingested with the food. Therefore, the body is deprived of nutrients to fight off cancer cells and free radicals.

Free radicals can damage the walls of the cells, cause DNA cross links, and structural damage to the mitochondria. These damages can lead to cancer cell changes and genetic mutation. Cancer cells are able to multiply uncontrollably and destroy neighboring normal tissues in the process. All of these destructive processes can be stopped if the tissues are provided with nutrients for repair. Nutrients also strengthen the immune system cells.

According to the Unified Field Theory, diseases and health problems originates from some form of malnutrition in a stage of life. This includes health problems that arose from genetic effects. All states of diseases, whether they are degenerative, infective, or congenital can be linked to nutritional factors as their cause and promotion. Disease elimination and prevention therefore, can be possible through proper nutrition.

Genetic Nutritional Requirements

Eating enables the body to extract nutrients from food when they enter the body's metabolic pathways. Nutrients from food are modified and molded by the body into molecules it can use. One of the metabolic pathways makes methyl groups, the epigenetic tags that silence genes. Some of the key components of this pathway responsible for making methyl are familiar nutrients like B vitamins, folic acid, and over-the-counter supplements. When a person's diet is high in methyl-donating nutrients, the gene expression of the body can be altered rapidly, especially when the epigenome is first being established during early body development.

Chemical compounds compose the epigenome. These compounds mark or modify the genome, telling it what, where, and when to do it. There are many types of cells in the body with different epigenetic marks which can be passed on to the cells as they divide, and thus transferred to generations. According to Dr. Elnitski of the National Human Genome Research Institute in the United States, less than 2% of the human genome makes up the functional sequences that encode genes. Other functional elements such as promoters, silencers, enhancers, and RNA-slicing signals are found in 98% of the genome. These elements perform important roles, such as the regulation of the temporal and spatial patterns of gene expression. Understanding normal cell functions is crucial in determining the cause of many diseases and their prevention.

The epigenome controls specific cells differential expression. When histones and their tails are modified by methylation, phosphorylation and acetylation, the compactness of chromatin and the positioning of nucleosomes on DNA are affected. The structure of chromatin is important in gene recombination and repair and other genomic activities. Chromatin structure changes are important in the silencing of some cancer genes. Histone deacetylase inhibitors have been found to have anticancer effect.

In multicellular organisms, the cells have the same genetic instruction sets from nominally identical DNA sequences, even if their terminal phototypes are different. The basis of epigenetics is the non-genetic cellular memory responsible for recording environmental and developmental cues.

A pregnant woman's diet can cause critical changes that a child will carry into adulthood. The same is true for the diet of an infant. In animal studies, it was seen that methyl-donating folate or choline deficiency during the late fetal stages or during early postnatal development have caused some regions of the genome to be under-methylated when the animals reached adulthood. In adults a diet deficient in methyl still results in decreased DNA methylation but the effects are reversible when a normal diet is resumed.

Studies showed that additives and chemicals entering the body can also affect the epigenome. When yellow pregnant rodents were fed a compound found in polycarbonate plastic called BPA or Bisphenol A, the mother gave birth to more yellow unhealthy babies than normal ones. The rodent's exposure to the compound during early development decreased the methylation of the gene. However, when a group of yellow pregnant mice were fed foods rich in methyl, the babies came out a healthy brown. Supplementation of the mother's diet with nutrients counteracted the BPA exposure's negative effects.

BPA is used in manufacturing human plastic consumer products such as tin cans and water bottles. In 2008, controversial reports about the safety of BPA were published, so many merchants discontinued selling these products and products with BPA components.

Human epigenome formed from the womb throughout life may provide people the information needed on how to eat better. This is the basis of the field of nutrigenomics. Nutritionists look at an individual's methylation pattern and use it as a basis for a personalized nutrition plan. Medical practitioners will soon be able to understand their patient's disease by studying their family health history.

The technological advances in the field of molecular and recombinant DNA led to further studies in genetics and DNA sequencing and an understanding of the uniqueness of each individual due to genetic variations. Pharmacologists applied the effects of genetic variation in the evaluation of drug metabolism and individual adverse reaction to drugs in development of new drugs. During the last few decades, medical practitioners, geneticists, physicians, and nutritionists have been studying the effects of gene-nutrient interactions and genetic variation in the management of chronic diseases.

The enormous implications of the new genetics have ushered in the era of nutrigenetics and/or nutrigenomics. Nutrition research now focuses on the management of chronic diseases and its prevention which can result from shared genes and shared environment of families. Studies have been undertaken to determine the contribution and interaction of genes and the environment in human individual development. Knowledge of susceptibility to health problems due to genetics will help those who are at risk for certain diseases as well as their individual responses to specific diets.

The importance of the ability to target specific dietary treatment in the clinical and economic consequences of people susceptible to high prevalence diseases such as osteoporosis, hypertension, coronary heart disease, and possibly cancer has been recognized. Continuing research and investments in various studies have resulted in genomic and technological findings showing the therapeutic benefits of diet in preventing and treating chronic diseases. The end result is the improvement of the quality of life by people all over the world.

In addition, understanding of human susceptibility to diseases due to genetics will help in identifying those at higher risk and find out their specific responses to diets. Therefore, diets and novel foods for specific individuals, whole families, and identified groups for mitigation and prevention of diseases can be developed. According to Simopoulos (2002), nutrition scientists will have a greater role in the 21st century in the establishment of nutrigenetics or nutrigenomics as a major nutrition discipline.

Genetic variation has been found to affect tolerances of food in subpopulations and is now known to influence requirements in the diet. This gave birth to the new field of nutritional genomics and to the possibility of health optimization and disease prevention by individualizing nutritional intake based on the genome of an individual. However, because the studies are still ongoing and interactions between the gene and diet are complex, genomic knowledge when applied to population-based dietary requirements is not without risk.

Currently, recommendations are targeted to prevent nutritional deficiencies in general populations. If genomic criteria will be included in the recommendations, there may be differential risk or benefit in fortification policies that may affect subpopulations. There have been efforts in identifying gene alleles that can affect utilization of nutrients through genetic variations identification.

According to Stover (2006), there are underlying molecular mechanisms in gene-nutrient interactions. Understanding genetic variation and nutrient modification is expected to be the foundation of nutritional interventions and dietary recommendations that can result in individual optimized health.

CHAPTER 4- DIFFERENT TYPES OF DIETS

Man has always understood the role of diet and nutrition as fuel for their body. The body naturally craved nourishment and regularly felt the need to eat due to hunger pangs. As man advanced forward in knowledge and technology, man learned about the beneficial effects of specific foods and the ill effects of deficiencies in nutrients, vitamins, or minerals.

Throughout the ages, men and women not only aspired for good health through diet and exercise, they also aspired for an ideal silhouette equivalent to the idea of desirability in a specific period. This has given rise to many types of diet to achieve that healthy, physically fit look of the moment, as ideal silhouettes change with the times. The types of diets are listed below except for the Paleolithic Diet which is treated separately. The list has been excerpted from the book written by Haas and Buck (2006) entitled Staying Healthy with Nutrition.

☐ Omnivorous

Omnivorous is the diet of most people worldwide where both animal and vegetable foods are consumed. This is the easiest type of diet to balance.

☐ Carnivorous

Carnivorous is the diet of animal flesh eaters. It is hard to find true carnivores as most carnivorous humans also eat plants and vegetables. Meats are high-protein food with different fat contents and iron which are essential for growth and tissue repair. Meat consumption however, should be supplemented with fiber, Vitamins B, C and E and various minerals from vegetable foods.

The human diet has been primarily vegetarian throughout history - humans eating meat only on occasions. Even today, this is true in many parts of the world. However, meat have been heavily consumed in the last century in developed cultures due to commercial production and slaughtering of animals for food and packaging them for ready availability in supermarkets and stores.

☐　　Lacto-ovo-vegetarian

The lacto-ovo-vegetarian diet is a modified vegetarian diet that does not include consumption of animal flesh but includes consumption of animal by-products like milk products and eggs. Other vegetarians limit themselves to being lacto-vegetarians because they are averse to eating unborn fowl. Some others find eggs okay but exhibits allergies or sensibilities to milk products. The Lacto-ovo-vegetarian diet is mainly composed of fruits, nuts, seeds, legumes, grains and vegetables.

When a diet is more vegetarian, the risk of common chronic diseases is reduced. Vegetarians enjoy a lower blood pressure and are not as problematic about weight compared to the meat-eaters. There is a low incidence of atherosclerosis, osteoporosis, heart disease, obesity, high cholesterol, hypertension, and cancer in studies conducted on Seventh Day Adventists, who are mostly vegetarians. In the study of countries' eating habits, the incidence of heart disease and coronary artery disease have been found to correlate with the respective population's intake of meat.

However, protein is needed in the diet, so the lacto-ovo-vegetarian diet is a recommended diet than a strict vegan diet because of its component protein, iron, calcium and vitamin B12 which the body needs.

☐   Vegan

The vegan diet is the pure or strict form of vegetarianism. No animal flesh is consumed or any other products derived from animals such as eggs, butter, cheese, ice cream, yogurt, or other milk products. Only plant-derived foods are eaten such as grains, seeds, nuts, vegetables, legumes, and fruits.

The vegan diet is not recommended for children unless a more balanced diet is overseen by the parents for their growing children. This situation is also true for pregnant and lactating females because they need higher intakes of nutrients. It is possible for children and pregnant women to adhere to a strict vegetarian diet but there is a high risk of deficiencies and possible future health problems. The vegan eater is oftentimes underweight in relation to his or her body size and low cholesterol levels.

While the vegan diet is high in fiber, there is a potential Vitamin B12 deficiency and low iron and calcium levels. Other nutrients that vegans must ensure they are getting in sufficient amounts are Vitamin A, Vitamin D, Zinc, and Protein; although many vegans are conscious on watching that they get enough protein.

☐   Macrobiotic

Macrobiotics as a philosophy of life came from Japan and has been shared by many teachers and authors including a feature in the East West Journal magazine. The diet has been adopted by many people in America and throughout the world.

Macrobiotic diets consist of mainly cooked foods as raw foods are considered difficult to digest as well as too cooling for the body. Less than 5% of the diet is made up of fruits, and even these are cooked. There is a minimum of animal products and they are limited to white fish. Eggs and dairy foods are avoided. The diet is almost vegan, although it consists of more nutrients and protein than a vegetarian diet.

A macrobiotic meal consists of more than 50% whole gains, such as buckwheat, rye, corn, barley, millet, whole oats, and brown rice. Breads and pastas are eaten only on occasions as most baked goodies and flour products are avoided. Vegetables, except members of the nightshade family such as eggplant, tomatoes, peppers, and potatoes make up 20-25% of the meal. Avocadoes, sweet potatoes, yams, and spinach are all avoided including herbs and spices such as cayenne, garlic, and onions as they are considered very stimulating. Fermented soybean products are eaten as well as sea vegetables, seaweeds, and beans. Soups and salads are part of the meal, as well as some exotic sounding foods and pickled foods to aid digestion.

This diet is seen as a good balance of yin and yang from Eastern philosophy viewpoint and is said to stabilize, nourish and heal. Because of the avoidance of high-fat foods, refined foods, sugars, and chemicals, the diet is considered to be a step forward towards a balanced and more helpful diet. The variety of foods make it sufficiently balanced with regards to nutrition. There have also been many articles supporting the theory that the macrobiotic diet is helpful in curing various diseases although there is not much scientific evidence to support the theory. However, it is known that arachidonic acid from omnivorous diets enables cancer cells to thrive; so the reduced production of arachidonic acid from a microbiotic diet can account for the claims of its many health benefits.

☐   Raw Foods

The raw food diet basically consists of eating uncooked foods which still contains all the vital elements from nature. It is thought to be the most healing and healthy for people with congestive maladies. Seeds, nuts, legumes, vegetables, and fruits are invigorated by the energy of the sun, water, and nutrients from the earth. The raw food diet also consists of sprouted seeds and beans as well as unpasteurized milk products. The main drinks are herb teas, fresh juices, and water. Breads and wafers are made from grain and sprouted seeds. Alcoholic beverages, processed foods, chemicals, and stimulants are avoided.

Although the raw food diet is considered a healthy one that provides vitality and nutrients, it is usually low in iron, calcium, and protein which can lead to future health problems. It is a good diet for losing weight and a good diet to try especially for people with an adventurous spirit, and those who want to cleanse their systems.

☐   Natural Hygiene

The natural hygiene diet is a diet of raw foods with occasional fasting that can help cleanse the colon. It is an ancient system that began with the Essenes, a tribe of Jewish scholars who believed in detoxification of the body, mind, and spirit in preparation for the coming of the Messiah.

The principle of the natural hygiene diet is based on clean living and freeing the body of waste and keeping it clean. The natural hygiene diet became popular in Germany in the 1930s with many followers in Europe and America since.

☐   Fruitarian

The fruitarian diet consists of only fruits - considered nature's true gift of nourishment. However, this type of diet cannot nourish the body on a long-term basis as it lacks some of the nutrients needed by humans to live. The B vitamins, magnesium, calcium, iron, and other minerals are deficient in an all fruit diet, not to mention very low protein content. Fruits do not have fats, although some seeds contain essential fatty acids. The fruitarian diet can be purifying and invigorating but only recommended on a short-term basis as its long-term nutritional value is considered poor

☐   Fasting

A true fasting diet is consumption of water - and nothing else. A fasting diet is done only for specific circumstances and should be undertaken under the supervision and guidance of a nutritionist or a physician. People undertake the fasting diet on a cleansing-purifying-detoxification process. Technically, it is not a diet, as no nutrients are provided.

Juice fasting is another form of fasting with some form of nutrients from juices, although it is still nutritionally deficient. The rest from eating solid foods will let the body decongest and process what the body has stored as fat. Juice fasting though, should also be done only on a limited period.

☐   Weight Reduction

There has been a lot of weight-loss diets published, tested, recommended, and eventually lost their popularity. There are dozens of new diets that become popular every few years as people always look for answers to achieve a trim figure, or a sort of cure-all for their ailments.

Weight reduction diets are designed to reduce calorie intake, restructure a person's eating habits, or include a special food that is supposed to burn fat. The formula for weight loss is basically eating food with fewer calories and then burning the taken calories with exercise.

☐   Warrior's

The warrior's diet is eating snacks or small meals every couple of hours in a day. The meals are simple, with simple foods such as an apple, a handful of sunflower seeds or almonds, celery or carrot sticks, crackers with fruit, or a bowl of rice with cooked beans. It is the consumption of small amounts of food to serve as fuel for staying energetic during the day.

The diet is called a warrior's diet because the individual always get the energy they need from the diet for ready action. When people eat big meals, or a variety of foods, they lose energy and feel sedated as the blood rush to the digestive systems, which is the opposite effect of the warrior diet. People on the warrior's diet are alert and energetic.

☐   Natural Food

The natural food diet is also known as the whole foods diet and is the original tribal or native diet of many cultures. The diet is derived from nature, gathered or captured from the surrounding areas or cultivated by the people themselves. Nature provided the foods; people used them directly and cooked them or ate them raw to feed the population. Most tribes and native cultures knew the proper mix of grains, seeds and legumes to obtain the protein they need for nourishment. Fish was another good source of protein, as wells wild birds and animals.

These days, more people are following the natural food diet with the emergence of the health food and organic food industry. Foods with additives are avoided as well as prefabricated and refined foods rich in chemicals.

☐   Industrialized

The industrialized diet is a trendy diet with consumption of refined foods such as refined white flour and white sugar. The foods contain preservatives and additives for a longer shelf life, and for safe packaging and shipping. This diet is compatible with mass production ideology and the modern fast-paced lifestyles or urban environments.

However, when refined foods of the industrial diet were introduced to various tribal cultures around the world, general health degradation was observed. There was an increase in tooth decay, incidence of cancer, cardiovascular diseases, and diabetes in the population. The story is contained in the book of Dr. Weston Price entitled Nutrition and Physical Degeneration: A comparison of Primitive Diets and Their Effects.

..

CHAPTER 5- THE PALEOLITHIC (HUNTER-GATHERER) DIET

The Paleolithic diet has been a resurging popular diet since the 1970s when it came to the attention of the general public due to the praise it received from some athletes. Its principles can be traced back to the diet of the most ancient peoples, the cavemen or Paleolithic humans and has been passed on to many tribal cultures throughout the centuries. These days, humankind that hunts wild game and gathers vegetables, fruits, seeds and nuts for food on a seasonal basis is almost extinct.

Anthropological studies and archaeological findings suggest that these ancient humans were healthy with strong bones and good body structures, without the problems of chronic degenerative diseases. They had a very active lifestyle as they devoted their days to hunting and gathering food. Their daily activities and survival techniques provide them with vigorous exercise.

A book entitled "Paleolithic Prescription" written by Dr. Eaton, Dr. Konner and Marjorie Shostak suggests that the modern diet should be more patterned to those of the hunter-gatherer era. They cite that much of the chronic diseases in our modern culture are due to the consumption of fats in large amounts, notably saturated fats, which were not common in ancient times as the fat level of wild and free range animals are much lower.

Grains cultivated in the modern way as well as eggs and dairy foods can be wholesome but are also the most common sources of allergens. According to the Paleolithic Prescription, refined foods should be avoided and that meat should be from those animals that are organically grown or from the wild like free-range poultry and fish. Foods that do not use chemicals during cultivation, raising and preparation should be the foods chosen and eaten.

The authors of Paleolithic Prescription suggest the today's modern diseases are the result of a mismatch of our lifestyle with our genetic makeup. The new and fattier foods are said to be the root cause of many chronic degenerative diseases. The prevalence of these chronic diseases suggests that the modern man have not yet adapted genetically to the domesticated production of meats, milks and vegetables that use additives and chemicals to arrest diseases in livestock and promote faster growth of animals intended for the market.

.

CHAPTER 6- ACHIEVING PEAK ATHLETIC PERFORMANCE WITH PALEO DIET

The Paleo Diet for Athletes is said to be the best way to maximize athletic performance. The diet revolutionized the sports world when it became popular. It can fuel the body by selecting foods that the body has been designed to eat. Our Paleolithic ancestors roaming the earth more than 250,000 years ago performed to live; our modern athletes live to perform. The ancient way of life was dependent on the strength, agility, speed, and endurance the people needed in the hunt for meat and in foraging for food. Their performance is the ultimate in athletic activities.

The Paleo Diet is eating the way our Paleolithic ancestors ate, to make us run stronger, live healthier, recover faster, and perform better. The Paleo Diet for Athletes is a nutrient-rich plan packed with branched-chain amino acids, the potent stimulants of the body in building muscles and its repair. Following the diet also leads to moderate weight loss and slimming while enhancing athletic performance.

The Paleo Diet for Athletes reverses the effects of blood acidosis and boosts the alkalinity of the body, thereby preventing muscle loss. It also optimizes the body's immunity with trace nutrients, enabling athletes to stay healthy and free from illness for the best performance. It shows individuals the best time for loading up on carbs and times muscle fuel for optimum performance.

The Paleo Diet for Athletes is a step-by-step guide on modifying eating habits before, during, and after a workout. The guide is critical in adjusting food consumption for a quick recovery after a workout, readying the body for the next workout, and for superior health condition everyday of your life. It is an athlete's bible for a lifetime of fitness, high-performance eating and optimum daily health.

Not Just For Athletes.

The Paleo Diet is not just for athletes as it focuses on natural foods. It has evolved into variations for athletes and for non-athletes that want to explore alternate strategies for keeping fit. The original diet is composed of strict guidelines for the foods to be consumed and those that should be avoided. Since the 1970s, dieticians, researchers, and physicians have made slight adjustments to the Paleo diet for the needs and individual requirements of specific populations.

The Paleo Diet is beneficial for the general population because it promotes consumption of strictly real, non-processed food. Its high protein content and fewer carbs are good for weight loss regimens. Reduced carb intake is good not only for weight loss but in promoting general health. The fruits, seeds, nuts, vegetables, and vegetable oils in the diet provide essential nutrients, unsaturated fat, and fiber need by the body.

The diet is alcohol free and low in salt, reducing the risk of heart disease and resulting in lower blood pressure. Organically grown vegetables, wild game and fish, meat from grass-fed animals, and other organic produce are nutrient rich foods with great taste and unsurpassed health benefits for athletes and non-athletes alike.

CHAPTER 7- PALEO DIET FOODS, DRINKS AND FOODS TO AVOID

Paleo Diet Foods include:

☐ Lean meats – lean beef trimmed of fat, flank steak, top sirloin steak, extra lean hamburger, London broil, chuck steak, lean veal, lean pork, pork loin, pork chops, lean poultry, chicken breast, turkey breast, game hen breasts.

☐ Eggs – six eggs a week from chicken, ducks or geese.

☐ Other meats – rabbit, or goat met, organ meats from beef, lamb, pork, chicken liver, beef, pork, or lam tongues, beef, lamb, or pork marrow, beef, lamb or pork sweetbreads.

☐ Game meat – alligator, bear, bison, buffalo, caribou, elk, emu, goose, kangaroo, Muscovy duck, New Zealand cervena deer, ostrich, pheasant, quail, rattlesnake, reindeer, squab, turtle, venison, wild boar, and wild turkey.

☐ Fish – bass, bluefish, cod, drum, eel, flatfish, grouper, haddock, halibut, herring, mackerel, monkfish, mullet, northern pike, orange roughy, perch, red snapper, rockfish, salmon, scrod, shark striped bass, sunfish, tilapia, trout, tuna, turbot, and walleye.

☐ Shellfish – abalone, clams, crabs, crayfish, lobster, mussels, oysters, scallops, shrimps.

☐ Fruit – apple, apricot, avocado, banana, blackberries, blueberries, boysenberries, cantaloupe, carambola, cassava melon, cherimoya, cherries, cranberries, figs, gooseberries, grapefruit, grapes, guava, honeydew melon, kiwi, lemon, lime, lychee, mango, nectarine, orange, papaya, passion fruit, peaches, pears, persimmon, pineapple, plums, pomegranate, raspberries, rhubarb, star fruit, strawberries, tangerine, and watermelon.

☐ Vegetables – artichoke, asparagus, beet greens, bell peppers, broccoli, Brussels sprouts, cabbage, carrots, cauliflower, celery, collards, cucumber, dandelion, eggplant, endive, green onion, kale, lettuce, mushrooms, mustard greens, onions, parsley, parsnip, peppers, pumpkin, radish, rutabaga, seaweed, spinach, squash, Swiss chard, tomatillos, tomato, and turnip greens.

☐ Nuts and seeds – almonds, brazil nuts, cashews, chestnuts, hazelnuts, filberts, Macadamia nuts, pecans, pine nuts, pistachios, pumpkin seeds, sesame seeds, sunflower seeds, and walnuts..

Paleo Drinks

The Paleo Diet drinks and beverages is mostly bottled and mineral water. Diet sodas can be taken in moderation because they may contain harmful sweeteners. Coffee may also be taken in moderation.

Alcohol drinks are allowed in moderation in the Paleo Diet in accordance with the following:

☐ Wine – 2 four-ounce glasses

Russell Dawson

☐   Beer – 2 twelve-ounce serving

☐   Spirits – 4 ounces

Foods To Avoid

☐   Dairy Foods – all processed foods such as dairy spreads, cream cheese, butter, low-fat milk, ice milk, ice cream, frozen yogurt, yogurt, whole milk, skim milk, powdered milk, non fat dairy creamer.

☐   Cereal Grains – barley soup, barley bread, processed foods made with barley, corn on the cob, corn tortillas, cornstarch, corn chips, corn syrup, millet, rolled oats, steel-cut oats and all processed foods made with oats, white rice, brown rice, rice noodles, basmati rice, rice flour, rice cakes and all processed foods made with rice, rye bread, rye crackers and all processed foods made with rye, sorghum, bread, muffins, rolls, crackers, noodles, cookies, doughnuts, cake, waffles, pancakes, lasagna, spaghetti, pasta, wheat tortillas, pita bread, pizza, flat bread, and all processed foods made with wheat or wheat flour, wild rice, amaranth, quinoa, buckwheat.

☐   Legumes – adzuki beans, broad beans, black beans field beans, fava beans, kidney beans, garbanzo beans, lima beans, horse beans, pinto beans, navy beans, mung beans, string beans, red beans, white beans, black-eyed peas, lentils, peas, chickpeas, miso, peanuts, peanut butter, sugar snap peas, snowpeas, soybeans, tofu and all soybean products.

☐   Starchy Vegetables – cassava root, manioc, starchy tubers, potatoes, French fries, potato chips and all potato products, tapioca pudding, yams, sweet potatoes.

☐   Foods with high salt contents – bacon, deli meats, cheese, salad dressings, condiments, hot dogs, ham, frankfurters, olives, ketchup, processed meats, pork rinds, pickled foods, salted nuts and spices, salami, sausages, smoked fish, dried fish, salted fish, smoked meat, salted meat, dried meat, canned meat, canned fish.

☐   Fatty Meats – bacon, beef ribs, chicken and turkey skin, legs, thighs and wings, fatty cuts of beef, fatty beef roasts, fatty ground beef or pork, fatty pork chops and pork roast, lamb roasts, lamb chops, pork sausage, T-bone steaks, pork ribs.

☐   Soft drinks, Fruit juices and Sweets – all sugary soft drinks, canned fruit drinks, bottled fruit drinks, freshly squeezed fruit drinks, candy, sugars, honey.

CHAPTER 8- SIMPLE PALEO RECIPES

Broccoli, Bacon and Cashew Salad

Ingredients

3 bacon rashes, remove the fat and dice

1 broccoli, cut into florets dice the stalk

½ cup cashews, toasted

1tbsp. oil

Instructions

Boil broccoli in water for 5 to 7 minutes or until cooked through. Remove broccoli from water and transfer into in a large serving bowl. Fry the bacon for 4 to 5 minutes until it gets crispy. Drain the bacon of excess oil and mix with the broccoli and cashews. Combine well and serve.

Cauliflower Carrot Herb Mash

Ingredients

3 medium carrots, chopped

1 cauliflower head, cut into florets

2 cloves garlic, minced

1 medium-sized sweet onion, chopped

1 tbsp. minced fresh thyme

1 tbsp. minced fresh rosemary

2 tbsps. olive oil

salt and pepper to taste

Instructions

Season and steam the cauliflower and carrots using a steamer basket and a large soup pot until soft. Test it with a fork after 10 to 12 minutes. Heat 1 tbsp. olive oil on medium heat and sauté the onion, garlic, thyme and rosemary. Season the mixture with salt and pepper to taste. Set aside. Use a food processor to process the steamed cauliflower and carrots together with the sautéed onion, garlic, and herbs with the remaining 1 tbsp. olive oil. When smooth, garnish with fresh rosemary and thyme before serving.

Cashew Chicken & Lemon Asparagus

Ingredients

2 chicken breasts, skinless and boneless

1 bunch of asparagus

¼ cup of cashews, chopped

1 clove of garlic

1 lemon

3 tbsps. olive oil

Instructions

Finely chop the garlic clove and mix with 2 tbsps. of olive oil. Brush this mixture into the 2 chicken breasts. Place the breasts on a baking sheet and sprinkle with chopped cashews. Bake the chicken at 350 for 30-40 minutes. Chop off ends of asparagus and separately brush with remaining olive oil and lemon juice mixture. Add salt and pepper to taste, top with lemon slices and bake for 20 minutes in a baking dish. Serve with the chicken breasts.

Pomegranate Arugula Salad

Ingredients

½ cup pomegranate seeds

4 cups arugula

¼ cup walnuts, chopped

2 tbsps. balsamic vinegar

3 tbsps. olive oil

Instructions

Combine arugula, walnuts, and pomegranate seeds in a large salad bowl. Mix the olive oil with the balsamic vinegar. Drizzle over the arugula mixture. Toss and serve.

Butternut Squash Soup

Ingredients

2 medium-sized butternut squash (peel, seed, and dice into small cubes)

1 onion, diced

2 tbsps. grapeseed oil

8 cups water or stock

Instructions

Caramelize the onion until golden brown in a large soup pot, using grapeseed oil. Add the cubed squash and cook for around ten minutes until soft. Boil the 8 cups water or stock separately and pour the boiling stock into the squash/onion mixture. Simmer the squash mixture for about ten minutes. Puree and serve.

Rosemary Apple Chicken

Ingredients

1 whole 2-3 lbs. chicken

4 sprigs rosemary

4 tart apples, core and slice

¼ cup balsamic vinegar

¼ cup olive oil

1 tbsp. sea salt

Instructions

Rinse and dry the chicken before placing it in a baking dish over the sprigs of rosemary. Mix the olive oil and vinegar and brush the chicken with it. Sprinkle the chicken with sea salt. Arrange the apple slices in the baking dish. Bake the chicken for an hour and a half at 350oC, until it is golden brown.

Tomato & Basil Salmon

Ingredients

2 salmon filets

2 tbsps. chopped fresh basil

1 cup quartered cherry tomatoes

1 minced clove of garlic

1 tsp. apple cider vinegar

1 tbsp. olive oil

Instructions

Arrange salmon on a baking sheet skin side down. Sprinkle the salmon with salt and brush it with olive oil. Bake at a 425 oC oven for 15-18 minutes. Mix cherry tomatoes, basil, garlic and vinegar separately. When salmon is cooked, top it with the tomato and basil mixture. Serve.

..

CHAPTER 9- PALEO DIET AND YOUR HEALTH, HOW TO LOSE WEIGHT

According to Teta (2012), the Paleodiet is the ultimate diet for fat loss, but so many people find it difficult to stick to it. She claims BCAA or branched chain amino acids have something to do with this inability to stick with the diet because people naturally crave dairy and starchy foods which are to be avoided in the Paleo Diet.

To satisfy the cravings for dairy and hunger for starchy foods, BCAA supplementation is recommended. In addition, BCAA supplements spare muscle loss as well as provide key elements in the metabolism of glucose. As such, it is claimed to be a key element in sustaining a low carb diet like the Paleo Diet.

The physiology of the body is complex and sometimes there are many explanations for body reactions. The Paleo approach is based on being metabolically flexible. The human body possesses the ability to burn carbs and fats efficiently.

The consumption of fruits and vegetables in the Paleo Diet are unlimited. Carbohydrates from these plant-based foods are of low-glycemic index, so the rises in an individual's blood sugar and insulin levels are slow and limited. When the levels of insulin and blood sugar in a body are excessive, they can result in Metabolic Syndrome diseases such as hypertension, high cholesterol, obesity, gout, and Type 2 diabetes. Because the Paleo Diet is high in protein, fiber and omega-3, it helps in the prevention of Metabolic Syndrome.

According to Cordain (2012), protein helps to increase the metabolism of the body and slow down one's appetite. Scientists found that lean protein greatly influences body weight regulation, health, and well-being. Protein revs up human metabolism twice as much as carbohydrates and fats and causes the body to burn more calories. It is also satiating, so people eat less when consuming lean meat. Cordain says that the Paleo Diet will make an individual's metabolism soar, shrink his appetite, and melt away extra pounds.

.. The approach of the Paleo Diet is based on the largest and oldest human trial ever, human evolution. The Paleo Diet has revolutionized the way humans think about nourishment and food. While it may look like one of those fad diets, many people think of it as a lifestyle.

The Diet mimics the unique diet to which the human species has been genetically programmed for. This eating program has not been designed by humans – not by faddists, diet doctors, or nutritionists – but by Mother Nature. It is based on the gifts of nature used by man wisely in his evolution towards enlightenment and knowledge.

The modern Paleo Diet is the result of extensive scientific studies on the way of life of man's Paleolithic ancestors and an examination of the quantities of food they consumed and the classes of food available to them during the period. The results of the research showed the advantages of their type of diet in the sense that the type of food they ate was what Mother Nature intended for people to eat.

The Paleo Diet consists of fruits and veggies that will make the body slightly alkaline. This will improve the acid-base imbalance of the body and reduce the risks of osteoporosis, hypertension, kidney stones, motion sickness, asthma, and stroke. In addition, the high soluble-fiber of the diet helps keep the gastrointestinal tract healthy; while the omega-3 fat content will help in the prevention of inflammatory problems.

The Paleo Diet is sustainable because it does not restrict eating habits as severely as other fad diets. It is considered a perspective shift, a more revolutionized approach to food. There are various options or variations in the diet. People who want to get fit, lose weight, or want overall health improvement will benefit from the Paleo Diet.

. The Paleo Diet, with its lean protein is good for the heart in addition to producing a slimmer figure. According to Dr. Bernard Wolfe (University of Western Ontario, Canada), high protein diets are more effective than high-carbohydrate, low-fat diets in helping to lower total bad cholesterol and triglycerides. Another researcher, Neil Mann (Royal Melbourne Institute of Technology, Australia) found that people who consume lean meat regularly have lower levels of homocysteine in the blood. Homocysteines are toxic to the blood and damaging to the arteries, making people prone to atherosclerosis.

Various researches have shown that high-protein diets like the Paleo Diet are beneficial to the body, reducing the individual's overall risk of heart disease. High protein diets have also been found to improve the metabolism of insulin, reduce the risk of stroke, and help lower blood pressure levels.

Paleo Diet And Weight Loss

The modern Paleolithic diet revolves around the idea that 'ancestral diets worked better for maintaining human health, when compared to dieting habits introduced after farming and other agricultural advancements entered the modern world.'

In regards to weight loss produced from this diet, many experts have commented that the frequency of Paleo-related weight loss relates to how people can't control their food consumption, which makes them gain more weight over time as a result.

According to some experts, ancestral humans developed the ability to store fat for longer periods of time, due to the lack of' food supplies on the Earth. These 'fat storage reserves' allowed early humans to have some kind of sustenance in-between their next meal, which took place between longer periods of time. This also developed their 'preference' for foods higher in calories and fat, which fueled the body in between long periods of 'starvation.'

In contrast to modern eating habits, people now have more access to more food during shorter periods of time. This caused many modern people to develop something known as a 'food reward,' or a sensation of pleasure 'achieved' when consuming foods of varying tastes and textures.

These sensations are mainly felt after consuming highly processed foods, which are likely filled with unhealthy and artificial calories and fats that disrupt the natural balance of consuming foods for nourishment.

Many nutritional experts, in fact, pin this phenomenon down on the loss of eating for nourishment. Now that many people 'eat for pleasure,' obesity as an epidemic has grown into a bigger problem over the past few years.

When it comes to losing weight on this diet, people immediately start seeing results, since this diet 'recreates' the natural food environment that early humans followed in the past. Using diets like the Paleo diet is a matter of learning how to lose weight in a 'sustainable way' that works best with the body.

Many people start losing a good amount of weight when switching to the Paleo diet. Others may struggle, though pick up their progress once they get used to the program. The Paleo diet is designed to help people accomplish their goal of 'returning to their roots' to lose weight—no matter the pace they move.

The best way to lose weight and gain overall health is to eat a low-fat, plant-dominated, high-carbohydrate diet. For weight loss to happen, a net caloric deficit must happen. However, many people feel hungry and unhappy with low calorie, high carb diets. When they decide that they can't stick with it anymore, they usually go on a binge and rapidly regain the weight they previously lost.

The Paleo Diet is a better alternative because it is a high-fruit, high-protein diet with low to moderate amounts of fat. However, there is an increase in the quantities of monounsaturated fats and omega-3 that are beneficial to the body. The thermic effect of protein is two to three times that of carbohydrates and fat. It means that the diet revs up the individual's metabolism, so weight loss is speeded up.

In addition, protein from lean meat is much more satisfying to consumer than carbohydrate, so it makes one feel fuller and satiated sooner and much longer. Finally, the Paleo Diet is recommended because there are numerous researches and clinical trials that show the effectiveness of high-protein, low-glycemic load diets like the Paleo Diet in the promotion of weight loss and maintaining an achieved ideal weight.

.

REFERENCES

Brown, C. (2011, October 3). The Paleo Diet. One Result: Look Like an Athlete.   Retrieved   from http://www.oneresult.com/articles/nutrition/paleo-diet

Cao, G., Booth, S. L., Sadowski, J. A., and Prior, R. L. (1998). Increases in human plasma antioxidant capacity after consumption of controlled diets high in fruits and vegetables.   National Institutes of Health, U.S. National   Library   of   Medicine.   Retrieved   from http://www.ncbi.nlm.nih.gov/pubmed/9808226

Carrera-Bastos, P., Fontes-Villalba, M., O'Keefe, J. H., Lindeberg, S., Cordain, L. (2011, 8 March). The western diet and lifestyle and diseases of civilization. Dove Press Journal: Research Reports in Clinical Cardiology. 2. 215-235.

Cordain, L. (2012). AARP the Paleo Diet revised: lose weight and get healthy by eating the foods you were designed to eat. Hoboken, NJ: John Wiley & Sons.

Cordain, L. (2005). The Paleo Diet for athletes: a nutritional formula for peak athletic performance. Emmaus, PA: Rodale Books

Cordain L. (2002). Paleo Diet. New York: Wiley and Sons. 104-112.

Diet Generation. (2012, February 27). Home Page. Diet Generation: A Diet for the Weight   Loss Generation.   Retrieved from http://dietgeneration.com/

Dietary Fat. (n.d.). Nutrition for Everyone. Centers for Disease Control and Prevention. Retrieved from http://www.cdc.gov/nutrition/everyone/basics/fat/index.html

Eaton, S. B., Shostak, M., and Konner, M. (1989) The Paleolithic prescription: a program of diet & exercise and a design for living. New York, NY: Harper Collins.

Elnitski, L. (n.d.). Epigenome. National Human Genome Research Institute, National Institutes of Health. Retrieved from http://www.genome.gov/Glossary/index.cfm?id=529

Haas, E. M. and Buck, L. (2006). Types of Diets. Excerpts from Staying Healthy with Nutrition: The Complete Guide to Diet and Nutritional Medicine. Retrieved from

http://www.healthyshopping.com/books/cart.asp?ItemNumber=15876 11791

Joyce, C. (2010, August 02). Food for thought: meat-based diet made us smarter. NPR: the human age. Retrieved from http://www.npr.org/2010/08/02/128849908/food-for-thought-meat-based-diet-made-us-smarter

Kimball, J. W. (2011, September 24). Human Nutrition. Kimball's Biology Pages. Retrieved from http://users.rcn.com/jkimball.ma.ultranet/BiologyPages/N/Nutrition.html

Neil, B. (2009, April 27). The diet generation: Shock figures reveal the weight worries of our 11-year-olds. Mirror News Online. Retrieved from http://www.mirror.co.uk/news/uk- news/the-diet-generation-shock-figures-reveal-789717

Nimboonchaj, N. (2007). Part V – our new diet generation. Shvoong.com. Retrieved from http://www.shvoong.com/medicine-and-health/1691965-new-diet-generation/

Nutrition and the Epigenome (n.d.). Learn. Genetics: Genetic Science Learning Center, The University of Utah. Retrieved from http://learn.genetics.utah.edu/ content/epigenetics/nutrition/

O'Keefe, J. H., Vogel, R., Lavie, C. J., Cordain, L. (2011). Exercise like a hunter-gatherer: a prescription for organic physical fitness. Progress in Cardiovascular Diseases. 53: 471- 479

People for the Ethical Treatment of Animals. (n.d.). The natural human diet. PETA. http://www.peta.org/living/vegetarian-living/the-natural-human-diet.aspx

Press Association. (2010, February 16). By 2020, 80% of men will be overweight, study shows. The Guardian. Retrieved from http://www.guardian.co.uk/society/2010/feb/16/adult- obesity-rises

Price, W. (1948). Nutrition and Physical Degeneration: A Comparison of Primitive Diets and Their Effects. Price-Pottenger Nutrition Foundation.

Riddihough, G. and Zahn, L. M. (2010, October 29). What is Epigenetics? Science, AAAS Org. Retrieved from http://www.sciencemag.org/content/330/6004/611.short

Sam. (2012, November 6). 5 easy Paleo Diet Recipes. Weight Loss and Training. Retrieved from http://weightlossandtraining.com/5-easy-paleo-diet-recipes

Simopoulos, A. P. (2002). Genetic variation and dietary response: Nutrigenetics/nutrigenomics. Asia Pacific Journal of Clinical Nutrition, 11(86). Retrieved from http://apjcn.nhri.org.tw/server/apjcn/Volume11/vol11sup2/S117.pdf

Ssali, C. (1996). Unified field theory of disease and nutritional causation or predisposition. Sarafina Foods & Supplies. Retrieved from http://www.sarafina.nl/ UnifiedTheoryMariandina.html

Stover, P. J. (2006, February). Influence of human genetic variation on nutritional requirements. American Journal of Clinical Nutriton. 83 (2). US Nationl Library of Medicine, National Institutes of Health. Retrieved from http://www.ncbi.nlm.nih.gov/pubmed/16470009.

Teta, J. (2012). Surviving the Paleodiet by using BCAA. Metaboliceffect.com. Retrieved from http://blog.metaboliceffect.com/2009/12/10/surviving-the-paleodiet/

U.S. Department of Agriculture and U.S. Department of Health and Human Services. (2010, December). Dietary Guidelines for Americans, 7th Edition, Washington, DC: U.S. Government Printing Ofice. Retrieved from http://www.cnpp.usda.gov/publications/ dietaryguidelines/2010/policydoc/policydoc.pdf

World Health Organization. (n.d.). Unhealthy diet. Global Health Observatory: Risk Factors. Retrieved from http://www.who.int/gho/ncd/risk_factors/unhealthy_diet_text/en/index.html.

www.ingramcontent.com/pod-product-compliance
Lightning Source LLC
Chambersburg PA
CBHW070823290526
45795CB00002B/823